# URINARY TRACT INFECTIONS :

*Understanding UTIs complications*

By

DOROTHY K. HULBERT

# DISCLAIMER

Despite her efforts to be as precise and thorough as possible, the Publisher does not at any time guarantee or suggest that the contents of this report are correct due to the Internet's tendency to change quickly.

Although every effort has been taken to verify the content in this publication, the Publisher disclaims all liability for any mistakes, omissions, or other interpretations of the subject matter. Any perceived slights towards particular people, groups, or organizations are accidental.

Like everything else in life, there are no guarantees of income made in books with practical advice. Readers are advised to respond based on their judgment regarding their circumstances and take appropriate action.

This book is not meant to be used as a source of financial, accounting, legal, or commercial guidance. We strongly suggest all readers to consult with qualified experts in the disciplines of law, business, accounting, and finance.

This book is recommended for printing for ease of reading.

**TABLE OF CONTENTS**

# CHAPTER 5

# OUTLOOK/PROGNOSIS

# CONCLUSION

# CHAPTER 1

# URINARY TRACT INFECTION

An infection of the urinary system, which includes the kidneys, bladder, ureters, and urethra, is known as a urinary tract infection or UTI.

The likelihood of developing a urinary tract infection is higher in women. According to some experts, the lifetime risk of contracting one is as high as 1 in 2, with many women experiencing recurrent infections for extended periods. A UTI affects about 1 in 10 males at some point in their lives.

Infections of the urinary tract (UTIs) are brought by bacteria and other organisms that manage to get past the body's defenses. They may have an impact on the tubes that connect the bladder, kidneys, and other organs. UTIs are one of the most common kind of short-term contaminations in the United States, prompting more than 8.1 million visits to specialists consistently.

The urinary tractcomprises the upper and lower urinary plot. The kidneys and ureters make up the upper urinary tract, and the urethra and bladder make up the lower urinary plot.

UTIs have various names relying upon where they happen. For instance:

- Bladder contamination is called cystitis.

- A urethra disease is known as urethritis.

- Kidney contamination is called pyelonephritis.

Urinary Tract Infection (UTI) is a disease that influences part of the urinary tract. When it influences the lower urinary plot, it is known as bladder contamination (cystitis) and when it influences the upper urinary lot it is known as kidney contamination (pyelonephritis).

Symptoms from a lower urinary plot contamination incorporate torment with pee, successive pee, and wanting to pee despite having a void bladder. Symptoms of kidney contamination incorporate fever and flank torment generally notwithstanding the side effects of a lower UTI. Rarely the pee might seem bloody. In the exceptionally old and the extremely youthful, side effects might be dubious or non-specific.

## SIDE EFFECTS

Side effects of a UTI rely upon which portion of the urinary tractis contaminated.

**Lower tract UTI side effects**

Lower tract UTIs influence the urethra and bladder.

- **Side effects of a lower tract UTI include:** igniting with pee, expanded recurrence of pee without passing a lot of pee, expanded criticalness of pee, ridiculous pee, overcast pee, pee that seems to be cola or tea, pee that has serious areas of strength for a pelvic torment in ladies, rectal torment in men

**Upper tract UTI side effects**

Upper tractUTIs influence the kidneys. These can be possibly hazardous on the off chance that microscopic organisms move from the contaminated kidney into the blood. This condition, called urosepsis, can cause hazardously low circulatory strain, shock, and passing.

- **Side effects of an upper tractUTI include:** torment and delicacy in the upper back and sides, chills, fever, queasiness, regurgitating

**UTI side effects in men**

Side effects of an upper tract urinary contamination in men are like those in ladies. Although, men with a lower tract UTI may likewise experience rectal torment.

**UTI side effects in ladies**

Ladies with a lower tracturinary contamination might encounter pelvic torment. This is notwithstanding the other normal side effects.

**Normal UTI Symptoms and Signs**

The urine of most healthy, appropriately hydrated individuals shows up light yellow or clear and is almost liberated from the scent. It additionally makes zero torment or inconvenience to pass.

However, for most individuals who experience urinary tract contamination, that is not the situation. Instead, they will probably experience somewhere around one of the accompanying pointers:

**A predictable and compelling impulse to pee**

When your bladder and urethra are kindled, this sludges up the receptors that signals when you want to pee.

**Pain or burning while peeing**

Bacteria disturbs the covering of the urinary tract, which then, at that point, spikes irritation that can cause a disagreeable sensation.

**Passing just limited quantities of pee at a time**

UTIs can make the urethra enlarge, which frustrates how much pee is passed.

- **Cloudy pee**

It's imagined that shadiness happens because your body's white platelets have developed while your framework attempts to dispense with the culpable bacteria.

- **Strong-smelling pee**

Bacteria can cause an off-putting odor.

- **Red, pink, or cola-hued pee**

This demonstrates the presence of blood.

**Pelvic pain or pressure**

This is felt in the focal point of the pelvis and can impersonate the impression of swelling.

**A full inclination in the rectum**

This UTI side effect presents just in men.

**Passing gas in your pee (Pneumaturia)**

It once in a while happens when your UTI makes air to be passed with your pee.

**Mucus-or discharge-like urethral release**

This UTI side effect is more normal in men than ladies. Here, your bladder and urethra's regular bodily fluid is endeavoring to get the body free from germs.

**Incontinence**

Lack of bladder control is especially obvious in the older.

*At the point when the kidneys are contaminated, other recognizable side effects might include: Fever, shaking and chills, nausea and vomiting ,upper back, side, or crotch torment*

While it's been noticed that disarray in the older is an indication of UTI,, a 2019 report in BMC Geriatrics presumes that there's deficient proof associating the side effect to that determination.

**UTI Signs and Symptoms in Children Are Different**

UTIs are the second most normal kind of contamination in youngsters, behind ear diseases. Unfortunately, early side effects of UTIs in small kids are not always apparent. Sometimes, there are no UTI side effects by any stretch of the imagination, or your youngster is essentially incapable to verbalize the UTI side effects the individual in question is encountering. With regards to children under 2 years of age, guardians need to check out these indications of urinary tract contamination:

- Fever

A fever of 104°F or higher might be the sole side effect in children. It's additionally the most considered normal side effect of UTI during a child's initial two years.

- Jaundice

Up to 18 percent of children with drawn-out or deteriorating jaundice additionally have UTIs. At the point when jaundice happens one entire year after birth, it's a serious area of strength for a UTI.

- Fussiness

Poor taking care of or inability to thrive

SluggishVomiting or diarrhea

Crying while urinating

In the meantime, more established youngsters for the most part have comparative side effects to grown-ups, including urgency, overcast pee, and agony during pee. For youngsters who've proactively been latrine prepared, bed-wetting is likewise an indication of a UTI.

# CHAPTER 2

# REASONS FOR UTIS

While this might sound pretty despondent, you can decrease your riskof a UTI by keeping away from some of the causes.

1. **You eat a great deal of sugar**

Microscopic organisms that cause UTIs love benefiting from sugar, so you risk giving a dining experience to them at whatever point your sweet tooth strikes.

If you eat lots of added sugars and get a genuine flood in your glucose, you might wind up with a portion of that sugar in your pee. A few food varieties and refreshments, similar to espresso, liquor, and chocolate, can likewise disturb your sensitive urinary tract and intensify a current UTI.

2. **You have diabetes**

Research shows that if you have diabetes, you're bound to get UTIs. The expanded riskmight be connected with a compromised resistant framework, fragmented bladder discharging, or vacillations in glucose.

3. **You wipe from back to front**

Wiping off from back to front can move E. coli, the microscopic organisms that are behind most UTIs, from the rectal district to the urethra. The lesson of the story: Always wipe from front to back.

4. **You have lots of sex**

The more sex you have, the likelier it is you could get a UTI. That's because microscopic organisms might move to the urethra from the vagina and from the perineum, which is the region between your vagina and your rear end.

Remember that sex toys, oral sex, and butt-centric sex can all acquaint microscopic organisms with anybody's pee parts.

5. **You don't pee after sex**

The danger of getting a UTI shouldn't prevent you from getting it. In any case, that doesn't mean surrendering to the afterburn.

One straightforward method for cutting your gamble: Head to the potty after you've completed your cavort. You'll conceivably flush out the microscopic organisms that might have advanced into your urinary tract.

6. **You hold it excessively lengthy**

We as a whole are occupied, however not getting some margin to stir things up around town — and not simply post-sex — causes more damage than great. You don't want pee should sit in your bladder for significant stretches because microscopic organisms in there can duplicate assuming they stick around excessively lengthy. So don't hold your pee.

### 7. You're utilizing techniques for anti-conception medication

With regards to UTI counteraction, not all anti-conception medication strategies are made equivalent. Fortunately, just a single technique is related to UTIs: diaphragm

As a result of where the diaphragm sits, it comes down on the urethra, which could prompt an expanded risk. The uplifting news? There are a lot of other extraordinary conception prevention choices.

### 8. You're utilizing condoms

Hold up! Listen before you toss out your affection gloves. Although, you ought to continuously rehearse more secure sex, unlubricated condoms can expand the risk of UTIs, conceivably as a result of expanded disturbance to the vagina during sexual movement.

Furthermore, utilizing spermicide with diaphragms and condoms can expand your risk. Try greased-up condoms without spermicide or utilize unlubricated condoms with a non-spermicidal ointment.

### 9. You don't hydrate

Guzzling H2O will make you go pretty frequently. What's more, that is something worth being thankful for. At the point when you do this, the microscopic organisms get flushed out before they get an opportunity to snatch hold.

### 10. You've got a cold, the flu, or sensitivities

You might be enticed to revile your occasional sniffles, a cold, or the feared influenza for making your life significantly more hopeless with a UTI, however, these infirmities aren't the reason. The prescriptions you take to oversee side effects could be.

However they're the bomb at holding your runny or stodgy nose under tight restraints, allergy medicines and decongestants could make you go less by causing urinary maintenance.

### 11. You're pregnant

Pregnant ladies have a higher possibility of getting a UTI because the hormonal changes cause the bladder muscle to unwind, in this manner postponing discharging.

If you're pregnant, you may have a diminished capacity to fend off contaminations, so any UTI-causing microscopic organisms are bound to get hold.

# CHAPTER 3

# FORESTALLING FUTURE URINARY TRACT INFECTIONS

**Washing and Hygiene**

To forestall future urinary tract contaminations, you ought to:

- Pick sterile cushions rather than tampons.
- Change your cushion each time you utilize the bathroom.
  Do not douche or utilize ladylike cleanliness splashes or powders. When in doubt, utilize no item containing fragrances in the genital area.
- Take showers rather baths.
  Stay away from shower oils.
- Keep your genital region clean.
  Clean your genital and butt-centric regions when sexual activity.
- Urinate before and after sexual activity.
  Drinking 2 glasses of water after sexual activity might assist with elevating urination.

- Wipe from front to back after  utilizing the bathroom.

- Avoid tight-fitting jeans. Wear cotton-material clothing and pantyhose, and change both atleast once a  day.

**Diet**

The accompanying enhancements to your eating regimen might forestall future urinary tract contaminations:

- Drink a lot of liquids, 2 to 4 quarts (2 to 4 liters) each day.
- Do not drink liquids that disturb the bladder, like liquor and caffeine.

**RECURRING INFECTIONS**

A few ladies have rehashed bladder contaminations. Your supplier might recommend that you:

- Utilize vaginal estrogen cream if you have dryness brought about by menopause. Take a solitary portion of an anti-microbial after sexual contact.
- Take a cranberry supplement pill after sexual contact.
- Have a 3-day course of anti-infection agents at home to utilize on the off chance that you foster an infection. Take a solitary, day-to-day portion of an anti-infection to forestall contaminations.

**Here are some home solutions for UTIs:**

**1. Wipe accurately**

Perhaps the best thing to do to forestall UTIs at home is to remain as spotless and dry as could be expected. Wiping off from front to back after peeing or a solid discharge will assist with holding microorganisms back from entering the urethra and going up the urinary tract.

**2. Wear cotton clothing**

Wear clothing produced using regular filaments to guarantee that the urethra stays as spotless and dry as conceivable to forestall bacterial section. Wearing apparel that is too close can obstruct wind current to the urethra. Without wind current, microscopic organisms can acquire a section and breed a climate that permits the improvement of a UTI. Wearing garments produced using filaments like nylon can trap dampness, permitting bacterial development.

**3. Try not to douche**

The presence of any microscopic organisms in the urinary tract doesn't mean the presence of contamination; "great" microorganisms are available and are significant for keeping a sound balance. Notwithstanding "terrible" microscopic organisms, douching can dispense with these "great" microorganisms and change your body's pH balance. Eventually, this might permit the "terrible" microscopic organisms to prosper. The vagina cleans itself bt utilizing release. If you want to clean up down there, utilize a pH-adjusted equation.

**4. Switch cleansers**

Your air pocket shower, body wash, and other cleaning items could be the guilty party to your UTIs. Utilize delicate equations that are color and aroma free.

**5. Change feminine cushions, tampons, or cups as often as possible**

Low-receptiveness cushions made of manufactured materials can open your vulva to microscopic organisms and increment your risk of contamination. Utilizing tampons can urge microscopic organisms to grow quicker, so it's essential to consistently change your tampon. If it pushes on your urethra and traps your pee, microscopic organisms can spread to the bladder. Changing the size or state of a feminine cup might help forestall intermittent UTIs.

**6. Stay away from spermicides**

Spermicide is a kind of conceptive prevention that is embedded into the vagina before sex to kill sperm. Spermicides might cause aggravation, eliminating regular obstructions of assurance from bacterial intrusion (and eventually contamination). Keeping away from spermicides while encountering a UTI is suggested. Furthermore, peeing previously and the after sex can assist with forestalling UTIs.

**7. Apply heat**

Having a UTI can cause uneasiness or torment in the pubic region. Warming cushions or hot water containers can assist with alleviating torment around there and are not difficult to utilize. Applying intensity to the pelvic region for around 15 minutes can have a major effect. Ensuring the temperature isn't excessively hot and that the intensity source doesn't straightforwardly contact the skin will forestall any aggravation or consumption. Scrubbing down might seem like an intelligent answer to ease UTI torment, however, most medical services experts exhort against bubble showers. If you do clean up, dispense with the cleanser and bubbles and limi the  time you drench.

**8. Hydrate**

One of the most mind-blowing home solutions for UTIs is to hydrate. Drinking a lot of water helps flush microscopic organisms out of the body. It's suggested that the typical sound individual beverage is somewhere around four to six cups of water daily.

**9. Drink cranberry juice**

At the point when microscopic organisms connect to cell walls in the urinary tract, this can cause urinary plot contamination. Proanthocyanidins, which are the dynamic fixing in cranberry juice, can assist with keeping microscopic organisms from connecting to urinary tract walls, which could assist with forestalling UTIs. Cranberry juice diminishes the quantity of UTIs an individual can foster for more than a year.

Drinking unsweetened cranberry juice to treat UTIs is exceptionally bantered in the clinical local area. While drinking the juice could help certain individuals, it may not work for other people. It's eventually dependent upon every person to conclude whether cranberry juice has a spot in the treatment of their UTI.

**10. Pee frequently**

Peeing frequently while encountering a UTI will assist with flushing microscopic organisms out of the urethra. Fighting the temptation to pee can keep microscopic organisms that are in pee caught in the bladder, which could exacerbate UTIs. Peeing before and after sex will likewise assist with limiting how many microscopic organisms that enter the urethra.

### 11. Eat more garlic

Consuming garlic is an extraordinary method for supporting your insusceptible framework, and garlic is notable for its antibacterial and antifungal properties. Allicin, one of the mixtures in garlic, has antimicrobial properties that have been demonstrated to be successful at killing E. coli.

### 12. Eat less sugar

Diet can be tremendous in the counteraction of UTI since it is brought about by a bacterial contamination. Microscopic organisms love sugar, so the more sugar you eat, the more you're taking care of the contamination.

### 13. Supplement with probiotics

Probiotics are enhancements of "good" microscopic organisms that assist with supporting a sound diaphragm and insusceptible framework. They can assist with holding destructive microscopic organisms back from prospering and help treat and forestall intermittent urinary tractcontaminations. The probiotic lactobacillus has demonstrated particularly compelling UTI counteraction for ladies.

### 14. Attempt homegrown cures

Uva ursi is a spice that has mitigating, astringent, and urinary disinfectant properties. Uva ursi has demonstrated to be compelling at treating and forestalling UTIs. It can be bought from wellbeing food stores and ought to be taken as coordinated by a nutritionist or medical services proficient.

Notwithstanding uva ursi, D-mannose is a sort of sugar that can assist with holding microscopic organisms back from adhering to the urinary tract wall. A few investigations show that taking D-mannose powder with water can assist with forestalling UTIs, particularly for individuals who get them as often as possible.

All homegrown enhancements ought to be taken in conference with a medical services proficient, as they might communicate with different prescriptions you are taking for different signs.

### 15. Utilize rejuvenating ointments with an alert

Oregano rejuvenating ointment is notable for its solid antibacterial properties. Studies have shown that oregano oil can be exceptionally successful at killing E.coli, however, it ought to be noticed that these examinations are for the most part finished in vitro — meaning in a lab utilizing logical strategies, not acted in people with contaminations.

Lemongrass oil and clove oil may likewise be a home solution for UTIs as a result of their antimicrobial properties, however, both have been contemplated against destructive microscopic organisms in comparative examinations as Oregano oil. Taking consideration before involving rejuvenating ointments as a treatment is significant.

# CHAPTER 4

# DIAGNOSIS AND TESTS

How are urinary tract infections (UTIs) analyzed?

Your primary care physician will utilize the accompanying tests to analyze urinary tract infections:

- **Urinalysis:** This test will inspect the pee for red platelets, white platelets, and microscopic organisms. The quantity of white and red platelets found in your pee can demonstrate an infection.

- **Urine culture:** A pee culture is utilized to decide the kind of microscopic organisms in your pee. This is a significant test since it decides the suitable treatment.

  If your contamination doesn't answer treatment or on the other hand, assuming you continue to get contaminations, again and again, your primary care physician might involve the accompanying tests to look at your urinary tract for infection or injury:

- **Ultrasound:** In this test, sound waves make a picture of the interior organs. This test is finished on top of your skin, its effortless, and ordinarily needs no arrangement.

- **Cystoscopy:** This test utilizes an extraordinary instrument fitted with a focal point and a light source (cystoscope) to see inside the bladder from the urethra.

- **CT examination:** Another imaging test, a CT filter is a sort of X-beam that takes cross segments of the body (like cuts). This test is significantly more exact than run-of-the-mill X-beams.

## MANAGEMENT AND TREATMENT

**How are urinary tract infections (UTI) treated?**

You should treat urinary tract infections. Anti-infection agents are prescriptions that kill microscopic organisms and battle contamination. Anti-infection agents are ordinarily used to treat urinary tract contaminations. Your medical services supplier will pick a medication that best treats the specific microscopic organisms that are causing your contamination. A few ordinarily utilized anti-infection agents can include:

- Nitrofurantoin

- Sulfonamides (sulfa drugs)

- Amoxicillin

- Cephalosporins

- Trimethoprim/sulfamethoxazole (Bactrim®)

- Doxycycline
- Quinolones (like ciprofloxacin [Cipro®])

You genuinely should follow your medical services supplier's bearings for taking the medication. Try not to quit taking the anti-microbial because your side effects disappear and you begin feeling significantly improved. If the contamination isn't dealt with totally with the full course of anti-infection agents, it can return.

If you have a background marked by successive urinary tract infection, you might be given a solution for anti-infection agents that you would take at the principal beginning of the side effects. Different patients might be given anti-infection agents to require consistently, daily, or after sex to forestall the contamination. Converse with your medical services supplier about the best therapy choice for you if you have a background marked by successive UTIs.

**What are the inconveniences of urinary tract infection(UTI)?**

Urinary tract infection can be effortlessly treated with anti-infection agents. However, if it isn't dealt with or on the other hand if you stop the prescription early, this sort of contamination can prompt a more serious disease, similar to kidney contamination.

**Could I at any point become resistant to the anti-infection agents used to treat a UTI?**

Your body can become acclimated to the anti-infection agents ordinarily used to treat urinary tract infection (UTI). This occurs in individuals who have exceptionally continuous contaminations. With each UTI and the utilization of anti-infection agents to treat it, the contamination adjusts and becomes more enthusiastically to battle. This is called an anti-microbial safe contamination. Along these lines, your medical services supplier might recommend elective therapies if you have continuous UTIs. These could include:

**Pausing:** Your supplier might recommend that you watch your side effects and stand by. During this time, you might be urged to drink a lot of liquids (particularly water) with an end goal to "flush out" your framework.

**Intravenous treatment:** In a few exceptionally convoluted cases, where the UTI is impervious to anti-infection agents or the contamination has moved to your kidneys, you might be treated in the emergency clinic. The medication will be given to you straightforwardly in your vein (intravenously). When you're home, you will be recommended with anti-infection agents for a while to completely dispose off the infection.

# CHAPTER 5

# OUTLOOK/PROGNOSIS

**What is the visualization (standpoint) for an individual with urinary tract infection?**

Urinary tract infections (UTIs) ordinarily answer to treatment. A UTI can be awkward before you start treatment, however, when your medical services supplier distinguishes the sort of microscopic organisms and recommends the right anti-microbial prescription, your side effects ought to improve rapidly. It's essential to continue to take your prescription for the whole measure of time your medical services supplier recommended. If you have continuous UTIs or on the other hand, if your side effects aren't improving, your supplier might test to check whether it's an anti-microbial safe contamination. These are more confounded contaminations to treat and may require intravenous anti-infection agents (through an IV) or elective medicines.

**LIVING WITH UTIs**

**When would it be a good idea for me to call my medical services supplier?**

Call your medical services supplier if you have side effects of urinary tract infection. If you have been determined to have a UTI and your side effects are deteriorating, call your medical services supplier. You might require an alternate treatment. Keep an eye out for these side effects specifically: fever, back pain, and vomiting.

If you have any of these side effects, or your different side effects go on after treatment, call your medical services supplier. A UTI can spread all through your urinary tract and into different parts of your body. However, treatment is exceptionally successful and can rapidly alleviate your side effects.

# CONCLUSION

UTIs are still a major burden for millions of people and our healthcare system, although they are frequently thought of as easily treatable illnesses. A significant obstacle to the therapeutic therapy of UTIs is the rising prevalence of antibiotic resistance among uropathogens.

If you suspect a UTI, it's critical to get medical assistance, especially if you also suspect a bladder infection or kidney infection, both of which are very dangerous illnesses.

Early urological infection treatment can reduce the risk of the infection spreading to the kidneys or bladder.

www.ingramcontent.com/pod-product-compliance
Lightning Source LLC
LaVergne TN
LVHW020544160826
845677LV00015B/4195

* 9 7 9 8 8 4 7 6 3 4 2 7 4 *